Meditation & Martini

The Subtle Cocktail of Balance

Meditation & Martini

The Subtle Cocktail of Balance

Dr Ranjit Rao

GYAN

ISBN : 978-81-212-1324-0

Price : ₹ 90

First Published, 2016

Published by

Gyan Publishing House
5, Ansari Road
Daryaganj, New Delhi-110002
Phones: 9811692060
E-mail: books@gyanbooks.com

Printed at: G. Print Process, Delhi.

Cataloging in Publication Data—DK
Courtesy: D.K. Agencies (P) Ltd. <docinfo@dkagencies.com>

Rao, Ranjit, author.
Meditation & martini : the subtle cocktail of balance / Dr Ranjit Rao.
pages cm
ISBN 9788121213240

1. Life. 2. Spiritual life. 3. Meditation. 4. Martinis. I. Title.

BD431.R36 2015 DDC 113.8 23

Contents

Introduction

This book is for those of you who want it all. It's for those who wish to enjoy everything the world has to offer materially, while simultaneously experiencing a full, healthy life of vitality that is spiritually vibrant.

If you wish to live the life of a monk or an ascetic, there are plenty of other manuals that you can turn to. Every path has its place and all of them are valid. This book is for the individual who is fully living in the hustle and bustle of worldly life. If you have a busy job, a hectic family life with a partner and children, and if you enjoy all the pleasures that life has to offer, such as food, alcohol, coffee, sex and friendships, and if you also wish to achieve the balance and inner peace of the Buddha, this book will offer you some insights.

Often the material and the spiritual seem poles apart. But are they really so different? Is it possible to be spiritually connected while in the midst of a cutthroat business deal, a life-saving surgery, or partying with friends? The answer is yes, and the way to do it is by experiencing your inner nature and establishing it as your ground-zero default state.

In the title of this book, *meditation* represents the spiritual, while *martini* represents the material, but don't take the title literally. I'm not trying to promote alcohol. As a surgeon, to do so would belittle the massive harm that alcohol causes in our society. There's no way that anyone can actually meditate while under the influence of alcohol. Meditation is about clarity, while the ultimate effect of alcohol is distortion.

The purpose of this book is to highlight that life can be lived with a certain balance and poise that provides a place for every experience. The only thing that must be given up is judgment.

Being a doctor and a surgeon has given me a unique view of life and the individuals within this rich tapestry. So many personalities, temperaments, situations, and circumstances, all reacting differently to the illnesses and challenges that life throws at them. While one person may be calm and philosophical about a new cancer diagnosis, another may be brought to their knees with paralysing fear. Every day, I am staggered by the courage and resilience that people display when threatened with a life-threatening problem.

Introduction

This book is a series of reflections on aspects of life that I have observed on my own personal journey, wearing a myriad of different hats: surgeon, doctor, yoga and meditation practitioner, spiritual seeker, student of Ayurveda, obsessive golfer, marathon runner, wine lover, husband, father, friend, and, most importantly, observer of the world around me.

I hope that some of these reflections will resonate with you on your own personal journey and help you make the choices that are in keeping with your own highest good.

I pray that all beings are showered with love and kindness, are free from suffering, make intelligent choices, and live their lives euphorically.

1

The Dilemma: Life, a Difficult Cocktail

Life does not come with an instruction manual. We are born into this world and grow up exposed to a host of different external influences. From this we come to a certain set of conclusions about life and what it means.

Life wasn't meant to be easy.

Nothing good comes without hard work.

Money doesn't grow on trees.

These are some of the well-known clichés that we have all heard while growing up. Generally the same paradigms get passed on from generation to generation, and the message can practically be etched into our DNA. Along the way we try to make sense of our lives and the world around us.

Many choices are available to help us rationalise our existence and dictate the way we live. Often we choose a pre-recorded paradigm that has been handed down to us rather than creating a tune of our own. The whole spectrum of possibilities exists in our minds, from the expansive and sometimes unrealistic 'anything is possible' to the fatalistic 'life is like this and we have no control'. What is important is that we arrive at a space where we are conscious choice-makers.

The entire New Age movement is based on the false premise that anything is possible. This is a ridiculous notion. If you're born a male, is it really possible to become a female? Only with surgery! But even then the genetics are still the same. If you jump off a building, is it really possible that you will fly? Not unless you have undiscovered superpowers. I rest my case.

Positive thinking will only get you so far. Like everything, it has its place, but it needs to be grounded in reality. I'm not suggesting that you shouldn't stretch your imagination as far as it will go, but the reality is that we are all born with a set of cards and our task is learning how to play our best game.

As a surgeon, I have observed many different programs within individual psyches. Optimism, pseudo-positivity, anxiety, fear, rigidity and depression are all distortions that may contribute to an illness, or cloud an individual's reaction to an illness. A classic example in my field of urology is prostate cancer. The media and various awareness groups have done much good work in raising the profile of this potentially deadly disease, but we do know that most forms of prostate cancer never kill and the disease simply requires careful monitoring. Some patients with an anxious disposition, however, who are faced with a diagnosis of low-risk prostate cancer are unable to accept non-treatment, and they sometimes end up on the treatment line suffering the consequences of incontinence, impotence and other problems.

At the opposite end of the spectrum are men with high-risk life-threatening prostate cancer who shun conventional treatment and try to cure their disease with meditation and herbs. While the exceptional miraculous cure may exist and be beyond the realms of standard measurement and validation, the vast majority of these patients miss the window of opportunity that treatment offers and end up succumbing to their disease.

Mental distortions cloud the ability to see

Mental distortions can often make it difficult for people to make the decisions they *need* to make rather than the ones they *want* to make. On the journey of life, how many people do you know who are well into their thirties, forties, fifties, sixties and beyond who are still trying to 'figure it' all out? Examine life carefully, and you'll see people around you who always have some drama going on in their lives while others seem to sail through life effortlessly. Although many will think this is just chance, in reality there are subtle patterns working behind the scenes that orchestrate the way life flows. Of course the circumstances we are born into, and the role models we are exposed to, can have a major influence on our way of thinking, but there still remains a choice in every moment as to how we respond to the situations around us.

Happiness is the starting point in life, not the destination

If a random sample of people were asked to define the purpose of life, many would say they consider happiness the goal, and they chase it in a multitude of ways. If asked, 'What do you want out of life?' many people would respond: 'To be happy.'

Accomplishment of goals is clearly an important aspect of a life well lived, resulting in a sense of achievement, satisfaction and happiness, but such happiness is often fleeting and short-lived. Once the transitory high has subsided, restlessness frequently begins to stir again.

To illustrate this point with a story, a wealthy businessman holidays on a remote island in the Bahamas. He sees a fisherman pulling in his net with a modest catch of fish. He approaches the fisherman and says, 'If I give you a bigger boat you can catch a whole lot more fish.'

'Why would I want to do that?' the fisherman replies.

'If you catch more fish, you can make more money,' the businessman responds.

'Why would I want more money?'

'With more money, you can buy a bigger boat.'

'Why do I need a bigger boat?'

The businessman, who is getting increasingly annoyed, says, 'With a bigger boat you can catch even more fish, make even more money, and employ people to run your business for you.'

'Why would I want that?' the fisherman asks calmly.

'Because then you'll have a huge fishing fleet with a global market across the world,' the businessman says, 'and you can relax.'

'But I'm already relaxed,' the fisherman replies. 'Why would I want to waste my entire life building up an empire so that I can relax, when I'm already relaxed with just one fishing rod and a few fish to cook?'

The businessman bows down to the other man. The fisherman was a sage in disguise.

Life is a little like this story. If you are taught from a young age that happiness is your nature, then the possibility of getting lost in a life of chasing shadows may never arise. Your life will then become an expression of happiness rather than a chase after it. You can hold a piece of gold loosely in the palm of your hand and enjoy its beauty, or you can grip it with tension and fear that it may be lost: same piece of gold, same hand, but two very different ways of existing.

You have a choice about how to live.

Clinging is a path to misery

Absolutely nothing in this material world is permanent. Trying to hold onto the elusive notion that life can be grasped and captured for eternity is a recipe for setting up tension.

If we examine the common scenario of boy meets girl, we see that attraction is based on many different facets of the other person, leading to a certain symbiosis of chemistry that ultimately forms a union. Whether the union is simply boyfriend/girlfriend, a flirtatious physical one, a more serious relationship where the two live together, or even marriage, possessiveness can strangle a beautiful union. Kahlil Gibran expressed this idea poetically and beautifully in his poem on marriage:

> You were born together, and together you shall
> be forevermore.
> You shall be together when white wings of death
> scatter your days.
> Ay, you shall be together even in the silent memory
> of God.

But let there be spaces in your togetherness,
And let the winds of the heavens dance between you.

Love one another but make not a bond of love:
Let it rather be a moving sea between the shores of
your souls.
Fill each other's cup but drink not from one cup.
Give one another of your bread but eat not from the
same loaf.
Sing and dance together and be joyous, but let each
one of you be alone,
Even as the strings of a lute are alone though they
quiver with the same music.

Give your hearts, but not into each other's keeping.
For only the hand of Life can contain your hearts.
And stand together, yet not too near together:
For the pillars of the temple stand apart,
And the oak tree and the cypress grow not in each
other's shadow.

When you are able to live with such trust, love and respect, your relationships and possessions become a foundation for growth rather than a restrictive hindrance. In the way that two mountaineers will use picks, ice axes and ropes to support each other in climbing Mount Everest, couples need to support each other in traversing the journey of life with all its cracks, crevasses and imperfections. Despite how it may seem on the surface, no one, not even a movie star, has the perfect life. We all have challenges to face, which have the potential to enable us to grow into better individuals.

A very important and subtle skill is the ability to *have*, combined with the freedom to *lose*. Imagine how freely you could live your life if you were prepared to lose everything you own and not be tainted or touched by the loss. Think about the things you hold most dear: health, family, house, car, money, reputation, friendships and occupation. If you were able to live your life according to your own unique life path, without a fear in the world of the consequences, imagine the freedom that would permeate your being.

Jim Carrey on life

Jim Carrey, actor and comedian extraordinaire, expressed this well when he said: 'I wish people could realise all their dreams and wealth and fame, so that they could see that it's not where they're gonna find their sense of completion.' A profound statement. If we all knew this from our childhood days, we would begin our lives with balance and perspective when it comes to finding happiness and contentment.

In the Vedantic (philosophical) tradition of India, this idea is defined as *svadharma*, which can be translated as the 'dharma' of the 'self'. *Dharma* is right action, and *svadharma* is the right action for the individual. The term 'right' is not used in a moralistic sense; rather, it is the necessary choice at any given moment. How do we know what is our *svadharma*? How do we know what the right choice is in a complicated situation?

Only an unclouded mind can know what is right and what is not. An unclouded or clear mind is one without distortions; a mind that can see things as they actually are without any projections based on fear or desire or other emotions. Some individuals are blessed with such clarity from a young age, but most of us have to work through some baggage to arrive at a state where the mind is settled enough to be able to see what is needed.

One of the most satisfying aspects of my work as a doctor and surgeon has been looking after our senior citizens. As people age they often gain perspective from life experience. Older people realise that being the richest man in the street is futile if their friendships and relationships have all collapsed and their children won't talk to them.

Working as a palliative-care doctor

As a junior doctor, I worked at Bethlehem Hospice in Melbourne. When patients arrived at the hospice, they knew there was only one way out. Most of them had a terminal cancer or end-stage organ failure, and were simply waiting for the inevitable, hoping that the end would be comfortable and the transition without undue suffering.

My job was to admit the patients, write up their drug chart, and formulate a plan after conferring with the consultant. This gave me the opportunity of taking a social and family history. I was genuinely interested in people's life stories; I wanted to know how they lived and how they were approaching death.

What became very clear to me was that in most cases each patient went through the dying process in a very similar way to how they lived. Those who had lived in fear generally died in fear, while those who had lived contented lives often died in peace. This was often, but not always, the case.

I distinctly remember a sister of the church, Francis Mary (name changed). She had terminal stomach cancer and was in constant pain, but she always had a smile on her face and a caring disposition. Every morning without fail she would ask me, 'How are you, doctor?'

I was at her bedside when she slipped into a coma. Her breathing became progressively slower and raspier, but at no stage did that pleasant smile disappear. I watched the rise and fall of her chest. Each time she exhaled, I thought it would be her last breath. She continued to take shorter and shallower inhalations, until eventually she stopped. Finally she was at peace. Everything became silent and I felt as though the universe had stopped to witness a great passing. I gazed at her face, marvelling that her serene smile had not diminished at all.

The game of life is a dilemma; how do *you* choose to play it?

The profound can be found everywhere, not just in spiritual textbooks. In the song 'The Gambler', Kenny Rogers sings:

You got to know when to hold 'em,
know when to fold 'em,
know when to walk away,
know when to run …'

The words of this song represent the choices you have, and making the best possible choices in any given moment. You may have no say in the cards you are dealt, but once you have those cards it's up to you to make sensible choices. How exactly do you do that? How do you integrate the perceived dilemma of the material life with its desire for wealth, possessions, name and fame, with the spiritual life and its properties of happiness, contentment, love and harmony? And can these two concepts really exist side by side, or is that just another empty promise made by modern-day soothsayers?

Only with a mind that is clear and free of distortions can you make the right decisions. Making the right decision doesn't necessarily mean that nothing will go wrong, but it will enable you to stay on the *dharma* or right path. According to the ancient Indian text, the *Bhagavad Gita*, 'It is far better to fail performing one's own dharma than to succeed performing someone else's dharma.'

This is a subtle thing and only you can know what's right. Not your parents, not the horoscope page, not the astrologer, and not the palm reader. It comes back to self-knowledge. Through observation, self-reflection, contemplation and meditation, your own truth will be revealed. Only then can you know whether you're making choices through the hazy lens of distortion or the clarity of wisdom.

Distortions scratch the lens of clarity

Anger, fear, inferiority, superiority, ego, external pressures, envy and cravings are all distortions that cloud the mind. I suggest you step back, self-reflect and start to observe the inner worlds. This is not esoteric airy-fairy stuff; it is very practical, and essential. As soon as you get it, it will be like turning on a switch. The switch of clarity will enable you to relax in the knowing that all is well; you have made the right choice, no matter what the eventual outcome.

Practical step 1

Grab a pen and paper and do your own SWOT (strengths, weaknesses, opportunities and threats) analysis. This is the first step towards living an integrated life, where the material and the spiritual can coexist seamlessly. Every new business needs a business plan, and similarly you need to take stock of where you are in your life, and where you want to go. Just like with a GPS, you need to write down your *current location* and *destination.* Only when you're clear about your goals can you make conscious choices between the various paths.

Strengths (internal)	1) ______ 2) ______ 3) ______
Weaknesses (internal)	1) ______ 2) ______ 3) ______
Opportunities (external)	1) ______ 2) ______ 3) ______
Threats (external)	1) ______ 2) ______ 3) ______

2

The Material: Martini

A martini is a magnificent drink made famous by James Bond, and epitomises opulence, luxury and decadence. To spiritual purists, the word *martini* represents the antithesis of spirituality. Is it really possible to live a life of extravagance and be spiritually centred, or are the two completely incompatible?

The first step is to realise that external situations have nothing to do with our inner state. We may have the simple needs of a monk, but choose to drive a Ferrari. Who are we to judge that a monk should travel only by foot and live a modest life? The material world poses many issues.

A family friend had completed his business degree and secured a job. It should have been a time of celebration, but instead he had fallen into the depths of depression. I asked him what the problem was.

'Now I'll have to wake up every morning and work from nine to five like my father,' he told me despondently, 'and do that for the rest of my life.'

This was the conclusion he had arrived at about life and the material existence.

In the material world, our sense organs are constantly uploading data from the external world to the mind, and the intellect within, in order to come to conclusions or judgments. These conclusions serve a very useful purpose when it comes to survival and safety. Take the example of fire. As children, we learn very early on that fire can be dangerous. We learn that it can be useful when it comes to cooking a meal or heating up milk on the stove, but that it also needs to be given due respect or we may be injured. Children learn these basic facts as part of their life skills in order to be safe from harm. Practical life skills such as these are essential to preserve our lives and prevent unnecessary accidents and injuries.

In a similar way, we come to a series of conclusions and judgments about the world around us. Often these conclusions lead to multiple compartments in our lives, and sometimes those compartments clash. For instance, the material compartment contains the desire to earn, enjoy and indulge, while the spiritual compartment suggests renunciation, withdrawal and isolation.

Is it possible to have a spiritual experience while living in the material world? And can you enjoy the fruits of the material world while living a so-called spiritual life?

The spiritual person may consider the person who is earning, spending, enjoying and indulging as unspiritual, while the material person will look at the spiritual person as incapable of enjoying the world around them. The capitalist makes fun of the socialist. The socialist mocks the environmentalist. The vegetarian judges the meat eater, and the vegan judges the vegetarian. The teetotaller proclaims that alcohol is the devil, and the drinker mistrusts the abstainer. And along the way, the quasi-religious end up in wars and kill each other in the name of their god.

The mind is the great classifier. Its role is to be constantly dividing, sorting and placing things in compartments. The role of the heart is to find unity, wholeness and connectivity. But by looking a little deeper below the surface and experiencing life in many different situations, it's clear to see that all these compartments are actually illusory.

You can be making a cut-throat business deal, performing a life-saving surgery or sweeping the floor, and have a transcendent experience that could only be described as spiritual. You don't need to be seated in the lotus position or on the yoga mat. Some may consider it blasphemous of me to suggest that the ephemeral can even be found on the dance floor of a rave party, sipping daiquiris in a lounge bar with friends, during the course of long-distance run, or skiing downhill.

This is not to suggest that alcohol, drugs, exercise or rave parties are paths to the spiritual; however, they do offer a glimpse into a state where all things are in unity and completely connected. This is the same state that yogis achieve through stilling the mind with yogic postures, breathing and awareness. Once the ripples of the mind come to a certain state of calmness, the underlying essence of unity can then be experienced.

The yogic perspective is to abstain from all things that may create mental fluctuations; hence, items such as alcohol, garlic, onions, meat, sex, and stimulants such as coffee or tobacco are considered against the objective of achieving mental stillness. Not everyone, however, is aiming for this degree of spiritual purity. For those who live fully in the material world and have objectives that include material *and* spiritual wellbeing, abstention from many of these things is not required. It's more important to bring gradual awareness into your life so you can make conscious choices rather than let your unconscious compulsions play out.

There is a Zen expression: 'Before enlightenment, chop wood, carry water; after enlightenment, chop wood, carry water.'

While the same activity may be happening on the surface, the underlying intention can be entirely different. It's up to each one of us to keep an open mind while we explore our own inner sphere.

I was recently at a surgical conference, enjoying a drop of Californian red with colleagues, when one of my friends said, 'I simply don't understand you.'

I could see that he was genuinely upset with me. 'Why, what happened?' I asked.

'On the one hand you meditate, practise yoga and speak of spiritual experiences,' he said, 'while on the other hand you enjoy having drink, driving a nice car, eating fine food, and you seem to be radiantly happy most of the time. What is it with you?'

I realised that he was annoyed because he was struggling with the dilemma of trying to be one or the other: spiritual or material.

I laughed. 'Loosen up, mate,' I said. 'Where do you get the silly idea that a spiritual person needs to be a certain way? There's no rule stating that to be spiritual you have to be deadpan serious and give up everything.'

The Vedas of India

The Vedas, a large body of ancient literature originating in India, offer guidance for those who live in the material world. The Vedas are a repository of knowledge gleaned by masters of great spiritual heritage who, having experienced the wisdom of the universe through silent contemplation and meditation, expounded many truths which they passed down from generation to generation. Even in modern times they still hold great relevance.

The Vedas describe the fourfold aims of life (known as the *purusharthas*) as follows:

1. Dharma
2. Artha
3. Kāma
4. Moksha

Dharma: right choices and path

Dharma is difficult to translate, but the literal meaning is to encompass that which is 'right'. It refers to the moment-to-moment choices that you make every second of your life. *Dharma* exists at every level of existence: as individuals, between individuals, within families, in our occupations, in society. It includes but is not limited to all laws that exist in society. It also includes our purpose in life, and the road map we use to express our best talents and learn the subtle meanings of life.

In every moment there is a choice. Sometimes these decisions are major, such as choosing a life partner or deciding on a profession, while at other times the choices may be as minor as deciding between eating an apple or a hot-chocolate sundae. *Dharma* determines what is the right choice. Neither apple nor hot-chocolate sundae is inherently good or bad, and both may be the right choice depending on the situation!

Sometimes *dharma* may seem very obvious while at other times it may throw the individual into total confusion. The graphic scene of the warrior Arjuna on the battlefield in the Hindu epic of the *Mahabharata* is an outstanding example of a confusing and difficult choice. Arjuna had to choose between doing his duty and fighting as a soldier, or killing his teachers, who were on the opposing side. Although killing might first appear to be against *dharma*, in this situation right action determined that he must fight. Arjuna was guided by Lord Krishna, a figure who represents divine guidance from the higher self or soul.

The lesson here is that we all have an inner guide that can be heard given the right conditions. In order to hear that guidance, the mind has to be brought to a state of balance. A mind that is clear, unruffled and poised is said to be in 'a state of yoga'. No matter what each person's path in life, it is entirely possible for the mind to become still and allow the underlying awareness to guide our actions.

The following story illustrates the concept of dharma, where the wisdom lies in making the right choice at the right moment.

When I worked as a junior doctor in a hospital emergency department, occasionally I had to deal with some situations that were highly embarrassing for the patients. A young lady came into the emergency department who had apparently been scratching her throat with a toothbrush when she 'accidentally' swallowed it. The entire toothbrush had travelled down her throat and food pipe into her stomach. I called the general surgical team down to see her.

With a straight face, the surgeon said, 'Look, we can either cut you open and remove it, or we can pass a telescope through your mouth and try to grasp it.'

The young lady was adamant that she did not want any treatment, saying she would instead try to pass it out in her bowel motions. For the next week she presented to the hospital for a daily x-ray to see the progress of the toothbrush. On the seventh day she developed severe pain; her bowel was perforated and required emergency surgery to extricate the toothbrush. Clearly she had made the wrong choice, possibly because her mind was clouded by fear of surgery or some other emotion.

Artha: acquisition of material possessions

Artha is the need, desire and requirement to accumulate material possessions. The acquisition of resources by right means is said to be following one's *dharma*. It is important to keep *artha* in perspective to avoid material abundance becoming our life's entire purpose.

The wise seers of years gone by realised that the problem was not so much the pursuit of money and material possessions but making the acquisition of these the sole goal in life, which is exactly what has happened to many. The more we possess, the more we desire. It's a never-ending cycle. The higher the level of debt, the more we have to work, and the more we have to work, the less time we have available for exploring life in its totality. The definition of the rat race is being trapped in a self-inflicted cycle from which we are unable to extricate ourselves.

What is the solution? The solution lies in the moment of choice and using the powerful force of the intellect to choose consciously, based on our assessment of the world around us. Will it bring greater happiness to live in a mansion as opposed to a comfortable house? Will the satisfaction of earning enough money to buy a sports car outweigh the fear of that car getting a small scratch or dent? Conscious, intelligent choice is the only solution, and this can only happen in a mind that is clear and balanced.

Scientific studies have been performed on individuals proving that beyond a certain level of material wellbeing there is no increase in happiness levels. It's clear that we all require enough to be comfortable. Adequate shelter, transport, clothing and food are all required in order to live life in a fulfilling way. The problem occurs when we don't know how much is enough and we start comparing ourselves to others, craving more than we need or are able to afford. Again, this sets up another one of those rat race cycles.

The balance between living within our means without compromising current levels of wellbeing while investing for future growth is a life skill that is not taught in the school or home. Many learn this lesson from a bad business experience or by investing in speculative stocks that turn sour.

It's the responsibility of parents and teachers to discuss with children the importance and relevance of material wellbeing. While possessions are important, they are not so important that we should compromise our peace of mind and wellbeing in a never-ending chase for more, bigger, best. The lesson is to enjoy possessions without being possessed by them.

This may seem a rather heavy message for children to learn, but it's an essential one when it comes to choosing a career and life path. In the ideal world, children will choose a path based on skills, talents and passion, but in the material world, parents and career counsellors often advise children to choose paths that simply lead to a fatter paycheck.

I'm not denouncing the importance of money. Money is essential for providing basic needs and enjoying life's comforts, and it can be used for the greater good of society through philanthropy and charity. Money is just a currency, and like any other currency it comes and it goes.

As Francis Bacon said, 'Money is a great servant but a bad master.' This is the fundamental problem. There is no issue as long as money is treated as a utility rather than pursued as a goal, and as long as our happiness and sense of identity are not tied up with wealth and possessions. If we can achieve that state, money becomes a neutral quality.

Kāma: the desire to enjoy pleasures

It's a very natural tendency to move towards things that give pleasure and away from others that cause pain. *Kāma* signifies pleasure, and the desire to seek and experience pleasure. The ancient seers recognised that individuals come into this world to experience and enjoy pleasures as part of the grand journey of life. The only caveat to the enjoyment of pleasure is that it be guided by *dharma* or right action.

Those who choose to get married are making an agreement with their partner to be faithful. Adultery in the name of pleasure is clearly contrary to *dharma*, and will ultimately result in pain.

I was working in the emergency department of a small country town when the triage nurse came over to me with a big smile on her face. 'We have a bit of a problem,' she said.

'What's happened?' I asked.

She directed me to a cubicle where the curtains were closed.

I entered the cubicle and found a man in his forties who had placed a brass ring around his penis as part of an unusual sexual practice. His penis was severely swollen and engorged due to the blood being unable to return because of the ring.

I went through the standard procedures to try and drain the blood, but after several unsuccessful attempts I told him that the only way to remove the ring was to use a special bolt cutter that only the fire brigade possessed. He gave the all-clear and I phoned the fire station to explain the situation. In they came with the big bolt cutters. Fortunately the story ends well. We were able to remove the ring and I never saw the man again, but I'm sure he learned a huge lesson from the whole experience.

Sexual desire is rooted strongly in our consciousness. Remember how tumultuous were the waves of desire when you were an adolescent and what happened to those feelings over a period of time.

It's a perfectly normal phenomenon for desire to be highest in our more youthful years and for that to wane naturally over time, but unfortunately we live in an era where society and the media have made sex to be the ultimate purpose of life. It's not possible to open a newspaper or glossy magazine, or turn on the TV, without noticing that the media is trying to exploit the seed of sexuality that lives within. From this is born a whole industry of anti-aging and sexual potency until death do us part.

The ancient seers wisely recognised that it was important to give sexuality a means of expression without turning it into the main purpose of existence. They were indeed wise. Every desire needs to be acknowledged, accepted and addressed, and neither given free rein to rule unchecked nor suppressed unnaturally. As long as sexuality is kept in its rightful place, it can be enjoyed without being allowed to be bigger than it needs to be.

The mind that is swayed by desire will clearly find it difficult to settle in order to meditate. It's important to be aware of the mind and present desires, but then learn how to satisfy them according to *dharma* and let them find their rightful place.

Time has a way of settling all of this in its own way, but by simply becoming aware of the movements of the mind and its contents without any judgement or suppression, we can slowly bring the mind to a more stable state.

Moksha: the ultimate purpose of life

Moksha is liberation. Liberation, *nirvana*, *samadhi* and enlightenment are considered the true purpose of life according to most spiritual traditions. What exactly is this revered state of nirvana? Does it really exist? And how do we get there? Do we need to renounce all worldly possessions in order to experience higher states of consciousness?

More than two thousand years ago, Prince Siddhartha, the Buddha, asked these same questions that spiritual seekers ask themselves now. As a prince, Buddha lived a life of opulence, but he became unsettled when he saw a dying old man. He realised that one day he would also suffer the same fate as the old man, and he slipped away from the palace in the middle of the night to pursue the question: What is the purpose of life? He gave up everything and was close to death from starvation when it dawned on him that renunciation of material possessions and food was not the answer. When he gave up the search, enlightenment arose.

Sometimes enlightenment is written and spoken about as a higher state of existence accompanied by bells, whistles, sounds, colours and revelations. The search for a spiritual experience through yoga or other similar techniques is actually no different from the pursuit of a high through alcohol or drugs. It's only the method that's different.

Experiences are not the 'main game' when it comes to *moksha*; rather, they are ways of getting sidetracked. The pursuit of *moksha* solely as a life path is for a select few. In some individuals, the desire for the material may have genuinely dropped away on its own as a natural consequence of life, while others may have been born without the need to acquire. Neither way is better or worse than the other; they are simply different paths. In the yogic tradition, the full-time pursuit of *moksha* is known as the path of *sannyas*, and such individuals are termed *sannyasins*. If the mind is full of desire, no amount of saffron robes or sacred ash can quell the waves within. The journey has to be a natural progression that comes from inside.

The majority of us will find it difficult to approach *moksha* as a single path, but eventually, when we are able to free ourselves of attachments, desires and the sways of the mind, we can move towards greater freedom. We are liberated when we can live in the world but not be part of the world, which can slip off us like water off a duck's back. Life then becomes a game to be played without fear or concern.

Creating a successful material life requires a fine balance of mental and intellectual clarity against a background of spiritual poise and equanimity. Developing this equanimity is one benefit of a regular meditation practice. Only with a settled mind and razor-sharp intellect can the best possible decisions be taken.

Practical step 2

Make a very clear list of what you wish to achieve in your material life over the next five, ten and twenty years. Keep your list handy, as we will refer to it in chapter four. Be very focused, but at the same time be realistic. There's no point writing down that you want to be a brain surgeon if you feel faint at the sight of blood, or your dream is to be a ballroom dancer if you have two left feet!

Use the SWOT analysis from chapter one to make these goals achievable, based on your individual talents, and include some of the following categories:

Career	1) ______ 2) ______ 3) ______
Relationship	1) ______ 2) ______ 3) ______
Family	1) ______ 2) ______ 3) ______
Children	1) ______ 2) ______ 3) ______
Health	1) ______ 2) ______ 3) ______
Fitness	1) ______ 2) ______ 3) ______
Money	1) ______ 2) ______ 3) ______
Car	1) ______ 2) ______ 3) ______

Possessions	1) ________ 2) ________ 3) ________
Sex life	1) ________ 2) ________ 3) ________
Travel plans	1) ________ 2) ________ 3) ________
House	1) ________ 2) ________ 3) ________
Sports	1) ________ 2) ________ 3) ________
Hobbies	1) ________ 2) ________ 3) ________
Philanthropy	1) ________ 2) ________ 3) ________

3

The Spiritual: Meditation

Since the hippy days of the seventies, when the Beatles took to meditation under the guidance of Maharishi Mahesh Yogi, to the positive-thinking era of Anthony Robbins and the quantum theory of Deepak Chopra, much has been written about spirituality. Each group or branch has its own perspective on spirituality and meditation. Each branch has its place and each individual must find their own path.

It's not necessary to change your entire life around to live a so-called spiritual life. There are so many misconceptions about meditation and spirituality, but if you take only one thing from this book, remember this: there is no one person, guru or organisation that holds the entire key for you. Ultimately, your own solution and salvation lies in your own hands.

One day a patient came into the hospital having lost twenty kilograms of weight. She went through every scan and test possible: CAT scans, ultrasound, blood tests, colonoscopy, gastroscopy. Everything came back normal. I was a first-year intern, and after all the tests were done I had the opportunity to talk to her.

'What's been happening in your life,' I asked her, 'that could explain your weight loss?'

I knew I was opening a can of worms, but fortunately it was the end of my shift and I was able to sit and listen. What she said highlighted some of the thoughts that exist in society about spirituality and meditation.

She opened her heart. 'I grew up in an environment where there was no discipline, restriction or boundaries. I was sent to an alternative school and was allowed to do whatever I wanted. When I finished school and started working in sales and marketing, I realised that I had to follow certain rules. In order to make progress in my field I had a relationship with a senior manager and was given promotions and pay rises. As I became materially more prosperous and enslaved to my manager, my happiness levels plummeted and I fell into depression. In order to cure the malevolent materialism that had crept into my soul, I decided to turn to a spiritual life.

'As I did this, I became more and more isolated. I became vegetarian, then vegan, and then I lived completely on raw food. I studied yoga and began practising advanced yoga breathing techniques without any proper guidance. I hated the person I'd become. The weight fell away from my body until I was literally skin and bones. Eventually, after twelve months of wasting away, my body started to protest at the starvation and my family brought me to hospital.'

People are drawn to spirituality for many reasons. This woman illustrates one of the many reasons why some people gravitate towards spirituality. Running away from problems, trying to cure depression and anxiety, managing stress-related issues, and frustration and discontent with normal life are some of the many reasons.

If you decide to embark on this path, it's important at the outset to have a clear understanding of spirituality and meditation so your actions are grounded in a strong foundation of reality. If you have taken to meditation to manage stress, to aid in the search for enlightenment, or to be more productive it's more than likely you have missed the point or been misled. Meditation may be a useful temporary remedy that enables you to get through life, but that's about all. This is not to belittle the usefulness of meditation in navigating your way out of problems, but only when 'true' meditation occurs will your life be truly transformed.

In ancient traditions, meditation practices were not imparted until the student had been though many years of rigorous discipline and training. Students had to be ready. In modern times, meditation and mindfulness are dished out like fast food and considered to be the elixir for every problem. The solution lies somewhere between the two extremes.

If you begin with a practice of quietening the mind (whether you call this a spiritual practice or not) these things will happen automatically. Stress levels will come under control, productivity will increase naturally, health will improve, sleep will be sounder and, most importantly, you will move one step closer to enlightenment.

The ancient yogic tradition described a very methodical step-wise progression to meditation; it's worth examining this and how it applies to the modern-day seeker.

The eight limbs of yoga

The term *meditation* is one of the most misused in spirituality. Yogic science describes an eight-limb path to meditation and liberation:

1. *Yama* (do's)
    - i *Ahimsa*—non-violence
    - ii *Satya*—truth
    - iii *Asteya*—non-covetousness
    - iv *Brahmacarya*—sexual abstinence
    - v *Aparigraha*—non possessiveness
2. *Niyama* (don'ts)
    - i *Saucha*—cleanliness of body and mind

ii *Santosha*—satisfaction
iii *Tapas*—austerity
iv *Svadhaya*—study of scriptures
v *Ishvarapranidhana*—surrender

These first two categories of *yama* and *niyama* may seem somewhat austere for people living in modern times. These scriptures were written more than two thousand years ago, in a different age. They remain fundamentally true today, but perhaps with a little more flexibility, less rigidity, and less seriousness in the overall tone.

Non-violence applies to thought just as much as it does to actions. Where you choose to be along this spectrum when it comes to food is entirely up to you. A vegetarian or vegan with violent judgmental thoughts can be more violent than a meat eater who consumes meat with an attitude of reverence, offering a prayer before consuming meat.

Truth must be tempered with non-violence. If your spouse looks terrible in the morning, it's probably better to keep your mouth shut than make an honest comment!

Non-covetousness refers to your attitude to others' possessions rather than whether you go as far as physically stealing. There will always be someone that has more or bigger or fancier than you. Letting petty jealousy for temporary pleasures will spoil your peace of mind.

Sexual abstinence seems rather harsh, unless someone is

living a monastic way of life and has deliberately chosen celibacy as a way of life. In modern terms, *brahmacarya* means being loyal to your partner, and not overindulging your sexual desire without restraint. It does not mean suppression of sexual desire, or unrestricted indulgence. It simply means letting sex take its rightful place: giving it enough attention, but not too much. It comes from an understanding that no amount of indulgence of any pleasure can bring ongoing fulfilment.

In Ayurvedic texts it is believed that the reproductive secretions carry the finest essence of energy called *ojas*, which is the culmination of the entire digestive process. Ayurvedic physiology states that digested food is transformed into plasma (*rasa*), blood (*rakta*), muscle (*mamsa*), fat (*medas*), marrow (*majj*), bone (*asthi*), and reproductive fluids (*shukra*). From *shukra dhatu* is formed *ojas*, considered to be the finest essence that supports the entire immune system.

This is difficult to reconcile from a Western medical standpoint; however, from an experiential point of view, what generally happens after the sexual act? Sleep. Once the energy has been dissipated, rest is needed. There may one day be modern scientific tests to measure *ojas* levels.

3. *Asana*—physical postures
4. *Pranayama*—breathing techniques
5. *Pratyahara*—withdrawal of senses from their external objects

The purpose of *asana* is not to be able to twist into a pretzel or to develop a taut backside. Physical postures, breathing techniques and detachment from external objects serve to stabilise the entire system. The Yoga Sutras of Patanjali state that *asana* is to be steady (*stutham*) and easy or comfortable (*sukham*). In essence, the purpose of *asana* is to enable the body to sit still comfortably with the spine erect. The breath is intimately connected with the state of mind. Observe yourself when you are relaxed are calm, on holiday perhaps, and compare this to the state of your breath when you're tired, angry or stressed. Yoga breathing techniques (*pranayama*) are used to consciously utilise the breath to create a certain state of mental stillness. Along with this, there will be a natural withdrawal from the sensory objects (*pratyahara*). Hence it is not a forced denial of external objects, but a natural progression to an internal state of quiet.

6. *Dharana*—concentration of the mind on a physical object
7. *Dhyanam*—meditation, an undisturbed flow of thought towards the object of meditation, with the act of meditation and the object of meditation remaining distinct and separate
8. *Samadhi*—oneness; there is no distinction between the act of meditation and the object of meditation

The last three, *dharana*, *dhyanam* and *samadhi*, are inward states of progressive concentration, focus and absorption. Only a mind that is calm and stable has the ability to move in this direction.

The act of sitting is not meditation. It's possible to sit with closed eyes and dream all kinds of things without ever coming close to a state of meditation as per the yogic view. This may seem like a semantic exercise, but any book on meditation needs to differentiate between what is a practice or technique, and what is meditation.

Before meditation can happen, the fundamentals must be right. For a seed to sprout and grow into a magnificent flowering plant, many things have to be taken care of first. The soil must be tilled. The seed must be watered. Sunlight and temperature must be conducive. Some of these things may be within individual control but some may be a matter of chance, or grace.

True meditation is difficult to achieve in the presence of stress about debt, chronic health issues, unemployment, or whether or not there is enough food on the table. Only once the foundation is established and settled can meditation become a possibility. This is a very subtle thing.

Unfortunately meditation does not function like a Band-Aid that will make stress disappear. It can be used in this way, but the true purpose of yoga and meditation is something much greater than that.

As long as you have this understanding about meditation, you can then choose to embark on a spiritual path with full awareness of where you are and what are your aspirations. Not everyone is aiming for nirvana or enlightenment, and that's absolutely fine. Most of us simply wish to have a mind that is happy and content most of the time and that is able to relax inwards when directed to.

Some spiritual traditions take an all-or-nothing approach, which may suit some individuals and temperaments, and it may even be necessary for a period of time if you wish to explore your inner world. As stated at the start of this book, there are different paths for everyone.

You may believe that you need to learn how to meditate because you're too stressed. You are correct in a sense, because there's no way that meditation can happen with a turbulent mind. The two do not go together, just like darkness and sunlight cannot be present at the same time.

The first thing that is required is a commonsense, practical approach to managing your mind and life better, so that things can settle down. Only once you have a stable foundation can there be any possibility of meditation. That's why, in yoga, the initial emphasis is on the ground rules, followed by stabilising the system with postures and breathing, both of which form a bridge to progressive inner states of stability and depth.

Sometimes when people embark on this spiritual path they will shun all that they consider material. This may be a necessary phase of spiritual unfoldment; however, once a reasonable level of awareness has been achieved, it will be possible to experience the subtle substratum that's always there. One need not be on the yoga mat in order to experience blissful states.

If you have ever had an experience where you were in a large gathering and been left in a rapturous state, or even tears, then you will have encountered something ephemeral in the midst of the mundane. It can happen while listening to your favourite singing artists, or absorbing the atmosphere at the MCG on Boxing Day, or enjoying an Australian rules grand final, or seeing a goal being scored during a World Cup soccer game. These are all examples of a collective heightened state of energy that can be best described as spiritual, or even ecstatic.

There's no need to run away to the Himalayas; however, it may be necessary to make some changes in your priorities and even the people you mix with while exploring these domains.

The first step is the very practical one of getting things settled in your regular life. Learn how to be sensible, practical, and how to live within your means. Learn how to make the right decision at the right place at the right time. After you've done all these practical things it will be time to take the next step.

Know the goal but focus on the flow

Life is a very subtle thing. On the one hand you need clarity of mind to make the right decisions to live your life in a sensible way, but on the other hand you have to keep in mind what the true goal of life actually is. Knowing the goal but focusing on the journey is a life skill. Yoga in daily life is not about bending yourself into crazy positions or having wild spiritual experiences. It's about creating a proper, stable foundation so that you experience the canvas on which your life plays out.

In ancient traditions there were numerous anchors that helped people maintain their focus and balance throughout the day, anchors that were tied to religious tradition. For example, in Hindu cultures the day would start with an invocation to the family deity, the lighting of the lamp and incense, and visiting the temple during the day. Even the auto-rickshaw driver in India today carries a small photo of their god and lights incense before starting the day—perhaps as the only way of maintaining any kind of peace in Indian traffic.

People living in Eastern countries often react very differently to the way we in the West react. For example, road rage is almost unheard of in India because people are experts in patience and waiting. For Westerners travelling in these countries, a level of patience is an essential requirement. Generally speaking, there is great inner stability and forbearance that seems to be hardwired into the consciousness of the East that has developed over thousands of years of their history. Western history, by contrast, is much younger and is still stabilising.

In modern life, a similar set of anchors can be created to help 'steady the ship' during the day.

As a surgeon, I utilise scrub time to centre myself, and pray that all goes well for the patient I'm about to operate on. Surgeons may perform operations to perfection, but the body still has to heal. Without that innate ability, every wound would fall apart, bleeding would never stop, and infections would go unchecked. I believe that my simple invocation ensures that all bases, seen and unseen have been covered for every patient. It may appear to be a superstitious action, but like every surgeon I realise that there are many factors beyond my control and it's my way of endeavouring to bring the best possible result for my patients.

For someone who receives and makes many phone calls during the day, it may be a process as simple as ensuring there is a pause of awareness every time the phone rings and every time a conversation ends.

For a businessperson who is going in and out of meetings, it may be just a few moments of attention to breath prior to and at the conclusion of every meeting. For a salesperson at a cash register, it may be a deep abdominal breath at the end of each transaction.

These actions all serve to bring the attention to a deeper, more stable centre where everything happens from a wider space of stillness, calm and love.

In Ayurvedic and yogic circles, it is well known that certain times of the day are conducive to meditative practices.

Anyone who has risen at dawn and heard the birds commencing their morning chirping will have experienced stillness in the environment. A similar kind of quietude occurs at sunset. These junctions between night and day, and day and night, are called *sandhya* (transition) and *vandhana* (salutation). We can all anchor ourselves at these more potent times of the day using any practice that brings the mind to a state of stillness and calm.

Transcendental meditation, which was popularised by Maharishi Mahesh Yogi and the Beatles, utilises a very useful analogy of dipping a cloth in dye and drying it in the sun. Each time the cloth is dipped, the cloth absorbs more of the dye, which then fades in the sun during the drying process. In the same way, in meditation the mind dips into the stillness of the self, imbibing some of those qualities, and with repeated practice the quiet, peace and stillness can become the nature of the mind also.

Stillness does not mean becoming inept, inert and impotent. When the need to act is there, you will find that you're able to channel the necessary energy in a far more focused and efficient manner—like a laser beam, rather than scattering the energy in a wasteful fashion.

Spirituality does not require turning your back on the world, but it does entail bringing greater awareness into your daily life. As this happens, the renunciation of more important things will occur automatically. Renunciation of anger, jealousy and fear will lead to a mind that is more stable and balanced. Renunciation of the need to have more, do more and be more will lead to an even greater sense of contentment.

The other side of the coin to renunciation is acceptance. Once you flip the coin to the side of acceptance, genuine peace, contentment and happiness is the natural result.

Often people who take to a spiritual path become very serious, in the same way that 'natural living' individuals become about health. There is a rigidity and fixed ideology that can go with both spirituality and health consciousness. When we are healthy, we usually take our health for granted. Often it's only when ill health strikes that we start to pay attention to ourselves. Whether it's the common cold, a severe bout of flu, a cardiac event, or a life-threatening cancer, these health crises can turn health into an obsession.

Examine the field of natural health, health and wellness, fitness, and spirituality and you may find many individuals who have an underlying sense of anxiety that is driving their health pursuit. If you're someone who is constantly ruminating about your health, fearing illness and disease, and scouring magazines and health-food stores for the latest longevity fad, you could be suffering from a condition that I have named H-RAD, or health-related anxiety disorder.

When does a healthy interest in physical and mental well-being and spirituality become a form of obsessive-compulsive disorder? When any activity becomes a preoccupation that prevents you from relaxing and enjoying your day-to-day tasks, the pursuit has become a disorder.

Every day in my clinical practice I see patients referred for a perceived physical complaint that can best be described as anxiety with a mask. Once the perceived problem has been explained as normal and nothing to worry about, the anxiety levels usually subside and the patient moves on. Sometimes the annual visit is nothing more than an anxiety-reducing consultation.

On many occasions, after I have assured a patient that they do not have prostate or bladder cancer, they will ask, 'But what if you're wrong? What if it actually *is* cancer?' It's almost as though these patients are willing themselves to develop the disease in order to have a genuine outlet for their anxiety.

I'm not suggesting that you take a complacent attitude towards health. Without good health, everything becomes tainted by the colour of pain and suffering, and it becomes difficult to enjoy even simple pleasures of life. Health and wellness is not something to take for granted, and you should strive for it by all means, but without turning it into an obsession.

The body, by its nature, is prone to problems. Despite the best efforts, every machine will have issues. Although your body is an amazing creation with an in-built system of intelligence that can fight cancers and infections, it may well succumb to some form of illness at some stage along your journey. The key is to combine a healthy dose of attention on wellbeing with an understanding that ill health can happen to even the most health conscious. It's important to recognise that anxiety may be underpinning an unhealthy obsession with being healthy.

It's interesting to note that when some of the longest-surviving communities are studied with respect to diet and lifestyle, researchers often make conclusions about diet, or single out micronutrients such as soy products or green tea, to explain the longevity. It's very difficult to measure these things scientifically, but could it be that such communities benefit more from their social cohesiveness and their relaxed dispositions than anything else? Could it be that people who are more relaxed, at ease with the frailties of the physical body, comfortable with their mortality, and who pay sufficient attention to their health without it becoming a full-time job are actually healthier?

Using the statistical bell curve as an analogy, it's usually the people at one extreme or another that run into health issues. People who suffer from diseases due to sedentary lifestyle, poor diet, and poor choices are at one extreme. These are the lifestyle diseases of modern civilisation, such as type-2 diabetes and coronary heart disease. At the other extreme are type-A individuals, who may be obsessive compulsive and workaholic in temperament, who often succumb to diseases due to what may be best described as stress.

The exception, of course, is sporadic, unexpected illness that can be attributed to bad genes, rotten luck or, in spiritual terms, *karma*. These are our dear friends and family, who out of the blue, have been struck down by illness. Only medical research with its intense study of genetics and molecular biology can find the solution for this group of illnesses.

Perhaps the solution, even with health, is focusing on the middle path, as the Buddha discovered. A little attention (but not too much) on diet and exercise, mental happiness and contentment, socialisation and friendships, savings and philanthropy, ambition and material comforts, and investing in the wisdom that all of this is ephemeral and transitory may well be the optimal way to live. It's impossible to conduct a randomised study that confirms this, but not everything in this world can be, or needs to be, measured.

Similarly, on the spiritual path the string must be tight enough to create beautiful music but not so tight that the string snaps. In this way, we can all have the humility to accept this life and cherish the time we have on our incredible planet.

Practical step 3

It helps to have a clear understanding about spirituality. Spirituality does not refer to how many hours you spend meditating, and nor is it something you can experience only on the yoga mat. Spirituality means being able to receive and share love in every single interaction, even the most mundane. Often there's a journey or path that leads to this ultimate experience, and it's important not to confuse the journey with the destination. In Eastern traditions, the spiritual practices are referred to as *sadhana*, and the culmination of the search is termed *moksha* or nirvana.

Too much focus on the destination creates unhappiness, whereas too much focus on the *sadhana* creates seriousness. It may help to write down the answers to the following questions:

1. What are my spiritual goals?	i) ______ ii) ______ iii) ______
2. What are my methods for obtaining these goals?	i) ______ ii) ______ iii) ______
3. By what parameters do I measure these goals?	i) ______ ii) ______ iii) ______

4. Would changing these goals affect my level of happiness now?	i) ____________ ii) ____________ iii) ____________
5. How would it make me feel if these goals were removed completely?	i) ____________ ii) ____________ iii) ____________

We will address these questions further along in the book, but for now it is useful to have an understanding about what you want; where you are and where you want to be; how you plan to get there; and whether it is really the destination you wish to travel to.

4

The Path: Balance

The New Age catchphrase 'Follow your heart' can lead to the erroneous belief that we can all be happy all the time. It's simply not possible. Contrary to the assertion that the heart, by virtue of its connection with the emotions and intuition, has a direct link to spiritual nirvana, there is nothing wrong with the rational, intellectual part of our being.

The nature of emotion is that it is in a constant state of flux. The nature of the heart is that it is emotional, holistic and intuitive. It's the seat of love and compassion. The nature of the head is one of intellect, pragmatism and analysis. A life lived with head alone, without heart, would be a very dry existence. Both have their purpose and place, and both need to be used at the right time and right place, in the right way.

Do you use head or heart?

When life choices are made purely from the heart, there's a very strong possibility that emotions will change and in turn change the path. What seemed like love in the beginning no longer seems the same two years later, and a change of heart occurs based on the ideology of following your heart.

On the opposite side of the scale, there are those in life who are brutally practical. They can seem almost heartless at times, apparently acting without any sense of kindness or compassion. If someone is required to run a business or do the accounting, a person who has strong analytical traits will be well suited to the task, although these people may need help in experiencing and expressing love and beauty.

We all come into this world with different amounts of head and heart qualities. The answer is not to use only one and shun the other. They both have very specific uses. It makes no sense to use your intuitive holistic side when deciding whether to pay your tax bill or a parking fine, but it's impossible to enter a relationship based on love, trust and faith by using only the analytical, logical part of the head.

The first gear of a car has a specific use, which is quite different to the reverse gear. Using the reverse gear to go forward simply does not work. Using the first gear to go one hundred kilometres per hour also does not work. As with a car's gearbox, the solution lies in knowing yourself, along with your specific traits, as well as knowing how well developed those faculties are.

Sometimes certain parts may need some work before they can function at an optimum level and be trusted in a real-life situation, which makes self-reflection and self-analysis crucial before making any important life decisions. Choices such as occupation, life partner and business decisions can impact your life in a huge way. It's always beneficial to take your time and reflect while utilising the correct 'instruments' to give yourself the best possible chance of making the right decision.

A sixty-two-year-old male patient came to see me regarding an elevated prostate blood-test result. After discussion about the implications and risk of prostate cancer, we proceeded to a biopsy. The results showed a high-grade aggressive prostate cancer, but fortunately there was no evidence of spread to lymph glands or bone. I recommended that we treat his prostate cancer aggressively, with radical surgery and possible follow-up radiation. Instead he chose to treat the cancer with herbal medicines and meditation. Within three months his prostate-specific antigen had risen to very high levels, and within six months he had metastatic disease in the bones. He passed away twelve months after the diagnosis. He had a very heart-orientated ideology that swayed him to a more gentle treatment option. There are times, however, when the situation requires compassion and gentleness, and there are times when it requires aggression. Although it's not possible to predict whether his outcome would have been different if he had chosen surgery, as the clinician I believe that it was a situation where there was a short window of opportunity for a successful surgical intervention.

Ideally the faculties of head/heart or intellect/emotion develop during childhood, and are established and integrated before formal adulthood. Most of us know children who are mature beyond their years, and have achieved that without much guidance or parenting, but more often than not, a certain level of guidance or moulding is required to help children reach this level of functioning.

Parents are in the unique position of being able to watch their children carefully in many situations, taking note of the youngsters' inherent strengths and weaknesses, and subsequently guide, encourage and support them to become fully integrated individuals with a mature and realistic understanding of themselves and the world around them. In order for parents to be effective, however, they need to have reached their own level of maturity, understanding and integration. Perhaps adults should have to take a 'parenting licence' before they're allowed to have children.

Children who are the unfortunate recipients of dysfunctional role modelling, unhappy households and poor parenting end up trying to unravel their issues for most of their lives, through no fault of their own. The best thing a child can be given is safety, security, stability and love to create within them the realisation that the world is a safe place in which to fully express their unique potential.

Whatever the background situation, a crucial part of life is reaching a state of self-actualisation so that you may fully express your talents and skills, while managing and strengthening your deficiencies or weaknesses.

No one can be one hundred percent correct all the time. Sometimes despite the best of intentions, planning and vision, things don't turn out the way you expect. This may be due to an error in your decision-making process, or simply an act of fate, both of which can teach valuable life lessons. If you find yourself in a difficult situation, try asking yourself what would be the absolute worst thing that could happen. The answer that comes to you will often give much-needed perspective.

In the words of Theodore Roosevelt: 'The best thing you can do is the right thing; the next best thing you can do is the wrong thing; the worst thing you can do is nothing.'

I have had many patients afflicted by cancer comment that cancer was the best thing that ever happened to them. It seems a most ironic statement; however, despite the pain, suffering and agony they face through the cancer journey, people often learn many valuable life lessons. Whether they achieve a cure or succumb to the disease, many feel they have learned a life lesson of monumental proportions.

A breast-cancer survivor in the United States made a comment about finding the 'can' in cancer. To her this meant that there was something good to be found within the difficult and devastating diagnosis of cancer. Many patients find that their perspective and philosophy about life changes, allowing them to deal and cope with their diagnosis, and that such a shift is beneficial for daily living also. It's often said that it's not what happens to us that matters, but how we deal with it.

Ayurveda and pragnaparadh

In Ayurveda, the ancient Indian holistic system of medicine, *ayur* means life and *veda* means knowledge. Hence Ayurveda is the science or study of life. According to Ayurveda, one of the causes of illness is called *pragnaparadh*. This can be translated literally as 'mistake of the intellect'.

When you know you're making the wrong choice but go ahead anyway, this is a mistake of the intellect. You realise that sugar is bad for your diabetes but you still choose to have a second serving of chocolate cake. You know that being angry with your children for a trivial incident is unnecessary but you still choose to become angry. Or you know that accepting a bribe for a business favour is an unethical action, but you still go ahead and accept it. These are all examples of *pragnaparadh*.

Pragnaparadh can be avoided by having a mind that is clear and a will that is unwavering. With an unclouded mind free of distortions and bias, the best possible choice at any given moment can be made. How that mind of clarity is created depends on each individual. There is no one size fits all. Every individual is unique and requires a different cocktail to function optimally.

A very physical person may require vigorous exercise, whereas a very analytical person may need to delve into the subtleties of philosophy to arrive at the same goal. While a ten-day silence retreat may suit one person, another person may require ten days of intense physical exercise. This fact allows every individual to chart their own way, depending on their own individual temperament, where they are in their life, and what methods they respond to.

Only the individual knows what they need. This is a refreshing notion for many people who wonder why they may not have benefitted in the same way as a friend or family member from various spiritual, yogic or meditation practices.

Types of meditation practices

When it comes to meditation, there are a huge number of techniques, practices and organisations that promote the practice of meditation. All of these are valid paths and can lead to greater states of mental clarity. If you're a meditation novice, I recommend doing some research to see what suits you.

Many techniques stem from religious or yogic origins. Some of them remain within those confines, while others have been neatly packaged by spiritual organisations. For those who prefer to remain outside the confines of a spiritual or religious cloak, the field of mindfulness meditation, while not suitable for everyone, provides an option for many.

Many of these spiritual traditions originated in the Indian subcontinent, which has specialised in exploring the human mind, psyche and consciousness. The following few pages give a brief description of some of the classical, modern, yogic and secular spiritual traditions.

If you are considering adopting a spiritual practice, assessing your own temperament and inclinations will make it easier to find the correct path. For example, if you are very intellectual in outlook you would probably not do well adopting a very devotional spiritual practice.

Traditionally in yoga, there are several broad paths that cater for different temperaments:

1. Karma yoga: the yoga of activity and action. The notion behind karma yoga is to do what's required without any attachment to the results. Selfless service is the best way to describe karma yoga.

2. Gnana yoga: the yoga of the intellect. In gnana yoga, the intellect is employed to lead the seeker to ask the question, 'Who am I?' By surgically separating and dissecting all aspects of ourselves that are not the 'I', we arrive at an intellectual realisation that we are neither the body nor the mind.
3. Bhakti yoga: the yoga of devotion. In bhakti yoga, the emotion is used to surrender to the object of devotion, which may be a god or guru. By subjugating one's ego, a merge occurs between the devotee and the object of devotion.
4. Hata yoga: the yoga of the energy systems. In hata yoga, the body, breath and mind are utilised to channel the life energies and enliven the entire energy system. It involves cleaning and purifying the system, and altering the way in which our energy flows.
5. Raja yoga: the 'royal' path of yoga. Raja yoga usually refers to the more inner contemplative and meditative aspects of yoga, such as *dharana*, *dhyana* and *samadhi*.

Broadly speaking, the various meditation traditions can be classified under one of four different groups:

- Classic spiritual organisations
- Modern/contemporary spiritual organisations

- World religions
- Secular movements

Classic spiritual organisations were traditionally started by a guru who had fully renounced the worldly life. Many of the messages are still applicable to modern times; however, the path of renunciation is for a select group of individuals who have no interest in worldly matters. Some of the founders and their groups include Ramana Maharishi from the Ramana Ashram, Swami Ramakrishna of the Ramakrishna Mission, Swami Vivekananda disciple of Swami Ramakrishna, Swami Chinmayananda of the Chinmaya Mission, and Paramahamsa Yogananda of the Self-Realization Fellowship.

Their disciples continue to provide spiritual guidance for seekers through books, classes and courses on meditation. These traditions are useful for those who have taken to a devout spiritual life, but equally to men and women in the midst of material life.

Modern/contemporary spiritual organisations generally stem from one of the great world religions, or from classic spiritual organisations. They are usually formed by a head, or guru, and the path varies accordingly. The iconic organisations of this class are the Osho group, started by Bhagwan Shree Rajneesh, and the Transcendental Meditation group, started by Maharishi Mahesh Yogi.

Transcendental meditation or TM became immensely popular after the Beatles visited Rishikesh during the hippy era of the seventies. TM utilises a mantra, which is a small sound that has no meaning. The mantra acts as a vehicle that takes the practitioner to quieter states within. To the credit of the organisation, much research was carried out on TM that validated its positive effects on parameters such as electrocardiography, electroencephalograms, heart rate and blood pressure. TM is sometimes criticised for being more expensive than many other meditation techniques, but the organisation believes it is important to give the practice value by putting a price on it. The science of mantra is described in the ancient texts such as the Rig and Atharva Vedas. Hence, this was not something that was newly invented; however, it was made available to modern-day people in a way that had never been done before.

Those in the Osho movement were known as the 'orange people' for their orange robes. Osho came under much criticism for his unusual methods, which included using sex as a path to liberation. He was a man of great intellect and was actually a professor of English before he came to the spiritual path. The Osho movement came to be characterised as a cult due to the blind belief and devotion the followers showered upon their guru.

There are many other modern and contemporary spiritual organisations, such as the Brahma Kumaris Foundation, Art of Living Foundation, Vipassana tradition, Isha Foundation,

Satya Sai Baba organisation, Mata Amritananda group, as well as the Hare Krishnas.

Each one has its slight difference. Some are guru based, while others place more emphasis on the actual practice. For example, the Brahma Kumaris and Vipassana movements are very much about the meditation practices, and their courses are completely free.

Organisations such as Art of Living, and the Isha and Mata Amritananda Foundations have a much stronger emphasis on the guru, which may lead to a guru–devotee-type relationship.

'Guru' literally means one who dispels darkness with light; in other words, one who helps to transform ignorance into wisdom. The concept of guru and disciple is a very interesting one to consider and it's worth spending a little time on the guru concept while working out which path to try. In the ancient traditions it was considered mandatory for anyone on the spiritual path to find a guru, and once they had done this it was important to dedicate themselves to the guru, who would then lead them on their path to enlightenment.

In every field of life, a teacher is required to help transform the novice into a competent and proficient person. Many people who have made great contributions to society have had mentors or teachers to help them climb the ladder of proficiency. It's very difficult to find someone who is truly self-made. Even those who claim to be self-made have studied the world around them and used examples to help mould their decision-making.

In the spiritual world, when does a teacher become a guru? The term 'guru' generally implies a sense of devotion, subjugation and subordination, where the disciple has chosen to believe in the guru and dedicate their lives to following their teachings. This path of surrender makes the decision-making process much easier for the seeker, whereby all conscious thought can be relinquished, and the teaching and instructions simply followed. A great element of trust exists in the guru–disciple relationship.

Although there are certain benefits in following a guru, the risk is that the individual foregoes all rational thought of their own. While this may be necessary when exploring more and more subjective fields that the meditator has no experience of, there are also potential dangers in handing oneself over completely to another individual or organisation.

The meditator must have a deep sense of trust that the guru's guidance is entirely for *their* highest good rather than the guru's. This of course works well when the guru has no other interest than the wellbeing of the meditator, but it becomes problematic when other motives come into play, such as financial scavenging, promotion of the organisation, or even sexual favours. Many spiritual organisations and gurus have been implicated in scandalous allegations, some of which have been true and others false. As with the doctor–patient relationship, there is a huge imbalance of power in the meditator–guru relationship, with much potential for abuse.

Similarly, a guru may abuse their power by manipulating their followers, some of whom may have experienced a minor spiritual experience. Once people have been indoctrinated with flawed beliefs, it's a very simple task to make them believe anything, and to justify their actions to themselves and others.

It's impossible to give hard and fast recommendations to those commencing a spiritual practice. While a guru-centric organisation may suit some individuals, it may be quite distasteful to others. It may even be detrimental to a person's spiritual growth. Ideally, prior to exploring the realms of the spiritual, it is important to establish a solid foundation. This foundation should begin with a healthy physical body, as well as an integrated and balanced emotional and intellectual system, so that sensible decisions are made at all times.

The purpose of yoga is to take individuals to a state where meditation happens spontaneously. Each group may have slightly different paths, but the ultimate aim is a state of 'oneness' (*samadhi*). With traditional yoga schools, although there may be a guru who heads the movement, there is rarely any requirement for the practitioner to become a devotee to the guru, as the teachings are simply those that have been handed down from generation to generation.

Some examples of these schools include the Bihar School of Yoga, Iyengar yoga, Krishnamacarya Mandiram, Sivananda

School of yoga, Baba Ramdev, and Patabhi Jois School of Mysore. Although there are many other yoga disciplines, such as Bikram or Ashtanga yoga, these tend to have a greater emphasis on the physical development of the body rather than spiritual unfoldment. Each has its place and it depends entirely on what the individual is looking for.

World religions include in their texts numerous stories of saints and sages who have explored the depths of meditation or danced in states of meditative ecstasy. Whether it is Hindu, Buddhist, Christian, Islam, Bahai or Jain, each has its own method and path to experience states of meditation. Examples include St Francis of Assisi and Shirdi Sai Baba who frequently went into rapturous states of meditation through their own religious practices.

Secular movements cater to the needs of individuals who prefer exploring meditation outside conventional religion and spiritual movements. Several other methods have become available, and currently the field of mindfulness meditation is experiencing great popularity. It is simple, non-religious, and its effects have been validated in numerous scientific papers and promoted by medical physicians. Other useful methods include progressive muscle relaxation and biofeedback.

The practice of mindfulness takes patience and consistency of practice, as there is no real 'anchor' for the practitioner to focus on apart from the breath. Breath awareness is a very effective practice, but it often takes time before the mind of a beginner meditator can settle enough to be sufficiently aware of the breath, and the more subtle movements of the mind and its thoughts. Frustration can occur early in the experience, where the practitioner simply says, 'I'm no good at meditation,' or 'I'm just unable to meditate.' It takes time to get to this level of proficiency; however, with proper and instruction and support, mindfulness can be a wonderful path.

The paths are many, but the goal is one

Despite what followers say, the method is not that important. What does matter is establishing a regular practice in order to learn how to still the mind. Once the mind learns how to settle easily, the inner stratum can be consciously explored.

The yoga tradition describes an individual as having several sheaths or layers: the physical body is termed *annamaya kosha*; the energetic system that drives the physical body is termed *pranamaya kosha*; the mental or emotional body is termed *manomaya kosha*; the intellectual body is termed *vignana maya kosha*.

What lies beneath these potential layers of turbulence is the *anandamaya kosha*, or bliss body. And beneath these and permeating through all of these is the *Atman*, which is the individual soul or consciousness—part of the universal soul or consciousness.

What we often refer to as 'happiness' is a superficial,

positive spike within the emotional body. Happiness is pleasant and enjoyable but short-lived, and often once the pleasurable sensation subsides, restlessness starts again till the next 'hit'.

Happiness that is more sustainable resides within the *anandamaya kosha*, or bliss body. An endogenous cannabinoid receptor called *anandamide* was discovered in 1992 and was named after the Sankrit word *ananda*. It's likely that some of the chemical neurotransmitters that are responsible for more sustained states of contentment, love, peace and harmony are somehow connected to the sheath called *anandamaya kosha*.

Ultimately, however, the purpose of yoga, meditation and all spiritual disciplines is the experience of the *atman*, or individual self, which is said to be *sat* (existence), *chit* (knowledge) and *ananda* (bliss) of the highest order. Despite this, not everyone needs to take up meditation to experience the ultimate. Many other benefits have been scientifically validated, and it is just as useful to start meditating to help establish some calm and peace, and some assistance with daily life.

Blending the material and spiritual

So much is written about work–life balance these days, which can be translated as material–spiritual balance, but the fact that we even have to discuss work–life balance, or stress management, is testimony to how badly we have managed our modern lives. Only once you look a little deeply into life and see what you have created can you appreciate what a comical situation existence is.

The solution is in finding the spiritual within the material, and simultaneously realising that the material is fully compatible with the spiritual. When you find the truth within the absolute mundane of material life while eating, mating, working, earning, parenting, drinking, indulging and dying, then all compartments disintegrate. These compartments of material and spiritual or work and life are self-created. Once you start to experience that there is actually no conflict between any of them, there is no longer a need for compartments at all.

For far too long the yogi has looked at the drinker with disdain, and the drinker has looked at the yogi with bewilderment. Each has something to learn from the other. When you can look beneath the surface from a place of deep love, it makes no difference at all what you are doing on the outside. Anyone, from any walk of life, can be just as spiritual as a meditator. Equally, a meditator can be just as violent as a murderer when their actions are motivated from a space bereft of love.

For most of us living in the hectic pace of the material world, what is required is enough attention on each aspect of our lives, combined with sensible decisions that allow us to continue to grow and unfold in a positive direction.

Practical step 4

- Identify ways in your day-to-day life where you can lift a task above the mundane and make it more spiritual, and show greater awareness.
- Identify ways in your spiritual life where greater grounding, solidity or even materialism may be helpful; for example, try to be less fixated on squeezing your meditation practices into the day.
- Observe areas in your life where you have become judgmental of others and work towards dropping the judging habit.
- List three people you have been trying to change whom you are now willing to accept as they are.
- Observe three aspects of your own life where you are prepared to revise or amend the way things should be.

5

The Traps: Cravings

I've seen far too many young people with incredible potential squander their opportunities and waste their lives in addictions, problems and mediocrity. Every year in Australian rules football, a talented youngster will come along and play amazing football, but then act irresponsibly after the game at a nightclub or pub and end up in a police cell. It's tragic at any level, and not just among elite sportspeople, to see a healthy young person with the world at their feet make a bad choice and end up in trouble.

During my time in medical school, a very bright and talented student who also played state-level baseball became addicted to marijuana. With the world at his feet, and within three years of becoming a respectable doctor who would contribute to society, he held up a petrol station with a fake gun and ended up in jail. He never went on to become a doctor, and I have no idea where fate took him.

Take care of your mind

As human beings, we all have weaknesses and frailties; that is the nature of being human. Our challenge is to take our talents and make use of them, while identifying our weaknesses and rectifying them. There's no doubt that the mind is the most important factor when it comes to health and wellness. All our actions stem from the nature of our mind. There's no point trying to give up marijuana or smoking, for instance, or any other detrimental habit, without dealing with the mind that is driving the desire.

Depression, fear, anxiety, obsessiveness, laziness, inferiority and poor self-esteem are all conditions that lead to poor decision-making and poor choices. It's possible that some people are born with a psychological tendency towards self-defeating traits, but for many it can be a result of the environment in which they have grown up.

The mind–body connection

A married male patient came to see me with debilitating pelvic and testicular pain. As a urologist, I find these conditions difficult to manage because there is seldom much that I can offer, apart from reassurance. There is generally nothing that the scalpel can fix.

After taking a full history, making an examination and checking the necessary tests, I reassured him that there was nothing seriously wrong with him. On more detailed questioning it became apparent that the problem started shortly after a trip to Asia, when he had had too much to drink and slept with a prostitute. He loved his wife and he was unable to cope with the guilt that had built up within him.

A caring ear to hear him out and a few sessions with a sexual counsellor relieved him of his burden, and eventually his pelvic pain lifted. He had seen his general practitioner, who had excluded all sexually transmitted disease. He knew he had made an error of judgement, and there was no reason to mention it to his wife and put her through unnecessary pain.

This patient was a classic example of the connection between mind and body: emotion and physiology. Countless studies have proven beyond doubt the link between mental stress and physical disorders. Depression and heart disease; anxiety and Crohn's disease; fear and obsessive-compulsive disorder have all been irrefutably linked.

More important than anything that can be learned in school, it is critical that teachers and parents observe their students and children well so they can help them conquer their challenges and strengthen their talents. The end result will be adolescents with a healthy self-esteem and confidence in their abilities, but with humility about the frailties of the human system, and the sense to ask for help from the right source when they need it. If they can achieve this by the time of graduation from high school, the chances are high that sensible decisions will follow.

It's when the individual grows up without the skills and resources to deal with their frailties that problems result. Once a problem spirals beyond a certain critical point, it can be nearly impossible to gain control again.

Being human is a humbling experience. We all make mistakes; we all get it wrong from time to time. A mature individual recognises their errors, takes full responsibility, makes amends as well as possible, and resolves not to make the same mistakes again.

Be aware of the traps

A person of maturity and wisdom sees the traps before falling into them. Just as in a video game, there are obstacles in life—common traps designed to bring people down—that we must try to avoid. There is a beautiful story in *The Tibetan Book of Living and Dying* about habits and the evolutionary process that occurs when changing or breaking habits. It goes like this:

'I walk down the street.
There is a deep hole in the sidewalk.

I fall in.
I am lost … I am hopeless.
It isn't my fault.
It takes forever to find a way out.

I walk down the same street.
There is a deep hole in the sidewalk.
I pretend I don't see it.
I fall in again.
I can't believe I am in the same place.
But it isn't my fault.
It still takes a long time to get out.

I walk down the same street.
There is a deep hole in the sidewalk.
I see it is there.
I still fall in … it's a habit.
My eyes are open.
I know where I am.
It is my fault.
I get out immediately.

I walk down the same street.
There is a deep hole in the sidewalk.
I walk around it.

I walk down a different street.'

Unless we have arrived at a state of contentment, these traps will almost always present as attractions. Money, name and fame are ways in which we can continue to grow, but those roads don't always lead to contentment and happiness. They can be false paths giving temporary happiness, eventually becoming a ladder leaning against the wrong wall.

There's nothing wrong with name, fame, wealth and power if they come about as a natural consequence of who we are as individuals, and according to our true life path. But craving and desire for them will only lead to unhappiness. These are the outward aspirations for people on the material path.

Those who are on the spiritual path often shun these goals in search of enlightenment. The truth is that there is no difference between the two ambitions; they are *both* ambitions but they have paths leading in opposite directions; one seeks outward accolades, and the other seeks inward enlightenment. If anything, spiritual ambition carries a heavier load of ego than does material ambition. The wise person will follow their own true path, and accept as a gift whatever comes as a result of that.

When a person of wisdom receives name, fame or money, they accept them as a responsibility to give back to society. There's nothing inherently good or bad about any of these aspirations, but it's the striving, together with the belief that they will bring happiness, that is completely erroneous.

The *traps* of fame, name, money or spiritual ambition are no different. They are one and the same. Understanding this fact will bring you immediate freedom. All striving will drop and contentment with the present moment will be what remains.

This does not remove the requirement to continue trying to do your best, and to continue trying to fulfil your potential. It simply allows you to see things as they really are; once you recognise that a trap lies ahead you will be able to negotiate it easily. More and more, you'll be able to sense the flow of where you need to go. Once you become aware of this flow, life can never be a struggle again. Synchronicity will start to happen around you because you will be flowing with the way things are meant to be.

This is not a fatalistic notion; it is an understanding that this existence is too complex and difficult to fathom. It is humility, and recognition that there's something much bigger than yourself—perhaps even a greater plan—and the realisation that you are a small part of this rich tapestry of life. When such a realisation occurs, humility will become a natural expression of who your really are. It's not pretence; it's as real as the air you breathe and you emit a fragrance of gratitude.

Spiritual ambition

In yogic and religious traditions *moksha* (nirvana, or enlightenment) is considered the ultimate goal of life.

It's a subtle point, but the important factor is the driving intention behind the pursuit. Does it come from a mature realisation of the world around us, knowing that ultimate fulfilment cannot be found outside ourselves? Is the focus on the process and unfolding rather than the destination? Or does the striving to be more spiritually advanced than others come from a place of insecurity or competition? In other words, what may appear as the same goal may have a very different driving intention.

You may read books on yoga, meditation, chakras, visions and enlightenment and fall into the trap of inventing hallucinations in the name of spiritual progress. Although some of these experiences may actually be real, they are not the ultimate goal and serve no useful purpose. A clear and mature vision will result in dropping the craving, letting go of any feverishness, and relinquishing the need to be in any space other than the one you're in right now. This vision will be grounded in a certain present-moment reality. It may not come with bells, whistles, or shining lights and chakras opening, *but* it's the only place to be. The rest will take care of itself along the way.

Drop the need for an 'experience'

One of the most dangerous aspects of organised religious and spiritual movements is that they can give the seeker a momentary 'experience'. It is seldom sustained, and often no sooner will a peak be experienced than the seeker comes crashing back down to earth.

In contrast, the yogic traditions follow paths in which the system is slowly strengthened and purified in such a way that the inner realms can be explored without risk of losing touch with reality. This is not a quick fix; it is a scientific process of steady work through body, mind and breath.

The spiritual experience in many unprepared seekers is actually no different to the drug seekers' experience, because neither of them lasts. The drug experience is stimulated by something from the outside, whereas the spiritual experience is triggered from the inside, but both end by coming down, and after coming down, the process creates the craving to go back up again for another high.

The solution is to drop the need for *any* experience, realising that the result will take care of itself in the long run.

Fear constricts; trust expands

There are so many different kinds of fear: fear of failure, fear of success, fear of humiliation, fear of rejection, fear of suffering, fear of causing pain. No emotion is more constricting to our life energies than fear. It literally causes the entire organism to shrink.

Breaking the fear tendency takes time, effort, compassion

and understanding, and the reality is that we're all going to make mistakes. We need to make the wisest decision we can based on our best level of understanding, then take one hundred percent committed action and let go of our attachment to the results.

As an avid golfer, I know that when I fear hitting a bad shot or missing a putt, chances are the result will be bad. But on days when I play with a carefree attitude and for the pure pleasure of the game, the shots are better, and even the scoring is optimised. With golf, it's important to have a good technique that's free of excessive tension. Life is no different. We need to have mental and intellectual processes in place that allow us to make the best possible decisions, such that the action and result are dissociated.

Every gardener knows that the only things within their control are creating the right soil, pouring on the right amount of water, hoping for the right amount of sunshine, and praying that the seed will take. There is faith that given the right circumstances the seed will germinate, but with the action of planting the seed, the possibility of failure also exists and the gardener has to be prepared for either outcome.

Worry, anxiety, fear and panic are often part of a spectrum of changes. Consider some of the things that immediately give rise to that deep visceral sensation in the pit of the stomach: dentists, doctors, injections, pain, illness, death and public speaking can all produce the whole range of symptoms within the worry-to-panic spectrum.

There are many things you can do to tackle the type of background anxiety that prevents people from living their fullest life. Writing down your anxieties and trying to understand why they may be irrational thoughts is an intellectual means of dealing with anxiety. Anxiety tends to be more emotive and visceral than intellectual, so as soon as your conscious mind has issued the instructions that everything is safe, your more unconscious, emotional and irrational side can start to play out.

Psychologists are professionally trained therapists who are able to analyse these symptoms more deeply, employing techniques such as cognitive-behavioural therapy to get to the bottom of any problem and create a permanent change.

Sometimes it is useful to incorporate worrying time into your schedule. During this time, allow yourself to worry as much as you like about anything, no matter how irrational. But when the timer stops, drop the worrying. One component of graduating to an adult, or mature, mind is learning how to let go of results. Focusing on what needs to be done in any desired situation and then surrendering the need to control the outcome is a very freeing feeling. This is both an inherent and a learned skill.

Some people do this quite naturally. *Total effort. Play to win. Not affected by the result. Keep trying under all circumstances.*

It takes a very integrated personality with a healthy self-esteem and a slightly thick skin to be capable of this approach to life, but this kind of confidence must be combined with clarity of thinking or else bullish behaviour will only cause collateral damage.

Most of us have to work on learning the skill of applying total effort without attachment to the result. It's very different to dropping the desire that many spiritual movements advocate. Without desire, nothing can happen. Desire is a very necessary impulse of the mind. But once the arrow leaves the bow, you need to understand that you have no control over the result. Your can control your preparation, training and firing of the bow. You can allow for external factors such as wind and humidity. But the ultimate result remains beyond your control, although your reaction to the result is *within* your control.

This is where participation in games and sports is essential for children. It teaches them how to participate fully and do their best, but more importantly it teaches them to be equanimous no matter what the outcome.

Judgement is more dangerous than junk food

You may have read a wonderful book by Robin Sharma, *The Monk Who Sold His Ferrari*. He writes about the corporate executive who sells his possessions in favour of spirituality. The reality, however, is that you can keep your Ferrari and be just as spiritual as a monk meditating in a cave. Again, it comes down to the intention you have towards the material object.

A materialist is one who is attached to the material. If you're sitting in a cave spending half your time meditating and the other half thinking of sex, drugs, and rock and roll, you're more of a materialist than the rock star who enjoys all of the above but without any need or attachment. You can have the Ferrari and live with the mind of a monk as long as you can be just as happy driving a bullock cart.

We need to drop any immature notions and stereotypes about what it means to be spiritual or material, and allow the two to intermingle naturally. When the CEO realises that the calm, laser-sharp mind of a yogi can assist his performance, and when a yogi realises that there's no obstacle to enlightenment by having possessions, many barriers start to come crashing down.

The purpose of *Meditation & Martini* is to show how the constructs of the mind are inherently flawed, and that by looking a little deeper we see that the spiritual and material can live harmoniously together in all facets of life.

Practical step 5

- Identify some of the traps that may be preventing you from being fully happy

- Ask yourself if your focus is more on the goal than the journey
- Identify any fears that are preventing you from living a full life

6

The Cycles: Eternal

In the environment, many cycles are readily apparent, such as day/night, and solar/lunar. The individual being as well as the whole universe is running in cycles. Cycles exist on a micro level as well as a macro level. The ancient Indian scriptures maintain that 'as is the microcosm, so is the macrocosm'. The same truth or reality can be approached from either angle. Now, more than ever, the yogi who explores inner dimensions is much closer to the astrophysicist who explores the outer dimensions. Descriptions by adept yogis of swirling energies on a canvas of dark emptiness sound like scientists describing lightning particles within a void held together by various forces.

When it comes to cycles, each one may support or hinder various activities. It makes sense from an efficiency standpoint to utilise these natural cycles or waves. In sleep, for example, a natural circadian rhythm or cycle determines when we should wake, when we should sleep, when we should rest and when we should engage in activity. Complex neuroendocrine hormones and neurotransmitters such as serotonin, dopamine and cortisol determine these cycles; however, they are also influenced by the sun; by light and darkness. Studies show that night-shift workers are more prone to depression, heart disease and diabetes than others who work during daylight hours.

Other obvious cycles include the physiological cycles that determine digestive efficiency, temperature changes that occur naturally, the female menstrual cycle, endocrine cycles of testosterone hormone in the male, and blood-pressure cycles.

Body temperature is lowest in the early-morning hours; melatonin is absent during the daytime and becomes detectable during dim light in the early evening; and testosterone levels peak around nine in the morning.

Ayurvedic physiological cycles

Ayurdeva describes the cycles of human physiology very clearly. All material existence is made up of the five elements—earth, water, fire, air and space—and these five elements combine to form the three doshas, Vata, Pitta and Kapha, which carry the qualities of the elements that form them. Vata represents the quality of movement, Pitta represents the quality of fire, and Kapha represents all that is stable. All three doshas are present in each person, but each one is dominant at a different time of the day:

Vata—2 am to 6 am
Kapha—6 am to 10 am
Pitta—10 am to 2 pm
Vata—2 pm to 6 pm
Kapha—6 pm to 10 pm
Pitta—10 pm to 2 am

Understanding and synchronising your system with the universal cycles can help you make choices that support your physiology rather than work against you. For example, if you're in the habit of waking up at 9 am every day rather than at an earlier hour, you will carry the heavier Kapha quality throughout your day.

The digestive system is collectively described in Ayurveda as the *agni*, the digestive fire, which encompasses all the secretions by the mouth, stomach, liver and gall bladder, pancreas and small intestine. Your digestive system functions strongest during the midday Pitta period, and so it makes physiological sense to eat your larger meal at this time.

With regard to sleep, it makes physiological sense to go to bed when the system is in the Kapha phase, before 10 pm.

We have all experienced the sensation of feeling sleepy, and then pushing though the tiredness and getting a second wind. This is because the body has entered the more active Pitta stage, which is the optimal time for the body to process and distribute the nutrients from the previous meal.

Getting out of rhythm for short periods of time will not have any deleterious effects; however, chronic poor patterns of daily living are likely to cause issues. In fact, Ayurveda considers prevention so important that it devotes several chapters in its main texts to daily routine (*dinucarya*) and seasonal routine (*ritucarya*).

With respect to seasons and different climate conditions, the body naturally seeks out certain foods, drinks, temperatures and qualities. For example, a cold, green leafy salad is more appealing on a hot summer's day than in the middle of winter, when a hot, hearty soup is more desirable.

Ayurveda is quite scientific about how it approaches seasons. During the cold months of winter, Vata (air/space) rises in the body. In order to keep balanced, the body automatically desires heavier and warmer food, hence the tendency to gain weight in winter. Once the temperature starts to warm, however, some of the Kapha (heavy) quality starts to liquefy, and we become more prone to colds.

Although this sounds simplistic compared to a Western medical model, it provides an explanation for why various conditions occur seasonally. Farmers who understand the environmental cycles know that in order for a seed to 'take', the soil needs to be well prepared. Ayurveda focuses more on the soil and creating a healthy physiology than the seed, or pathogen, but when a pathogen does break down the natural immune barriers Ayurveda has its own herbal armamentarium to treat the problem.

An exhaustive description of Ayurveda is beyond the scope of this book; however, good information can be obtained online, or by reading *Perfect Health* by Dr Deepak Chopra.

If you wish to live a life of balance, where the material and the spiritual exist simultaneously, a basic knowledge of the cycles can be very useful. Animals behave instinctively when it comes to eating, sleeping and mating, and perhaps do all of these with less fuss than human beings. Knowledge of food and hunger cycles can help you understand why a big meal before bed will result in a restless sleep, and why your body is much more prepared for digestion in the middle of the day. If you are planning to indulge, it makes sense to know when it's physiologically more suitable!

Sexual cycles

Sexual desire generally commences around the time when hormones kick in. It manifests through a heightened interest in the opposite sex, experimenting with self-play, desire for a partner, and engaging in sexual activities.

Those who have taken to a yogic or spiritual path often consider sex to be a hindrance. If one sits to meditate or perform yoga and unwanted sexual thoughts keep entering the mind, mental calmness and clarity can hardly occur. It's important to remember, however, that these are inherent, natural cycles that exist in all of us and to deny them would be to deny life itself. The sexual impulse varies from person to person, of course, as well as at various times of the month. Ayurveda notes that a person of Vata constitution may be highly excitable sexually, with a tendency to irregular and erratic sexual interest. A predominantly Pitta person may have a high sex drive, but with a tendency to dominate. And a Kapha person will have a slow and steady desire, needing a longer time for arousal but with stronger endurance.

It's more important than generally realised that couples are matched from the perspective of sexual desire. A Kapha female who takes a long time to become aroused and ready may be frustrated with a Vata or Pitta male who just wants to get the job done quickly. Similarly, a Kapha male with a low but steady sexual desire may not be able to match the sexual energy of a hot-blooded Pitta female.

In Western cultures, where societal norms are more relaxed, this kind of problem is quickly identified, and if incompatibility exists the relationship may end. In Eastern cultures, where arranged marriages were prevalent for a long time and still exist in some countries, many factors are taken into account when considering a potential alliance. Even astrological predictions that are based on the time of birth take note of a person's nature and predilections, and the aim is to match the two individuals on every level, including sexual desire.

Although the West has sorted out sexual compatibility well enough, unfortunately it has made sex a much bigger deal than it needs to be. Simultaneously, it has become mired in religious ideas of guilt and sin, which lead to a different kind of revolution—witness the sexual revolution of the sixties with flower power and sexual liberty for all. What was once a sacred exchange of love and intimacy between two consenting individuals has turned into a deep-seated requirement for more, bigger and better. The media, of course, portrays the false illusion that couples are having sex for breakfast, lunch and dinner, in all corners of their homes, with longer endurance and bigger orgasms, making the rest of the world feel inadequate and inept.

A thirty-year-old male patient came into see me one day complaining of problems with his erections. When I questioned him, he told me he believed his troubles stemmed from excessive masturbation as an adolescent. I reassured the young man that it had nothing to do with masturbation, and explained that almost all adolescents go through the process of masturbation and learning about their own sexuality. Somewhere along the way he had been given the false notion that masturbation is bad or wrong, and that if he continued he would suffer from the consequences. The real problem was that he was in a new relationship, stressed out at work, and unable to relax sexually with his partner and enjoy the mutual exchange of intimacy.

The truth is that life is never what it seems. The first step is to know ourselves, including our own sexual tendencies, which we should accept as real and valid rather than denounce as wrong, bad or sinful. Understanding that sex is just a small part of our lives helps to put things in perspective. Finding a partner who matches us sexually will enable us to express our sexuality during that cycle of our lives.

As we get older, often the emphasis on sex decreases naturally. In saying that, I have met many octogenarians who still have vigorous sex lives that remain an important part of their relationship. Overall, however, the importance of sex usually reduces with age, and companionship and friendship become the predominant features of many relationships.

For those who have taken to a more spiritual trajectory in life, it's even more important to know where and how sexuality sits within them. Denying the sexual impulse will only lead to an inner revolt, heightened desires and even sexual perversion. The group of individuals that take to *sannyas*, or monkhood, where celibacy is a requirement should first be sure that the sexual desire has been finished with. Only once that state has been arrived at will the individual be truly suited for a monastic lifestyle.

In Ayurvedic texts, the four stages of life are clearly described—student, householder, forest recluse, renunciation—and they are suitable for the vast majority of individuals. Only after student and married life, when all desires have been fulfilled and have run their natural course, is the mind ready for any inward contemplation.

That's not to say that if you are living the material life you shouldn't learn from spiritual teachings. Studying spiritual truths can provide balance and help you maintain a clear focus on the ultimate purpose of life. Ultimately, the only truth is to know yourself, and to live life accordingly, rather than trying to follow any preconceived notion about how you should live.

Karmic cycles

Delving into philosophy and spirituality takes us to the topic of *karma*. The word *karma* is now well known to the West, having been used in Hindu, Buddhist and yogic philosophies. It has come to represent the sentiments expressed in the saying, *As you sow, so you reap*, and, more plainly, *You get what you deserve. Karma* is the irrefutable law of cause and effect.

There is nothing overly spiritual about cause and effect. It is a law of physics in the material world. Every action you perform has an effect. In fact, every action you choose to perform is with the aim of producing a desired effect. When you choose to go to work, you expect a particular result in terms of goals, and, equally, you expect a paycheck for your work. This is a very practical and tangible example of *karma*.

Also on the physical and emotional plane but somewhat subtler is the effect of thoughts and emotions and the resultant physical chemicals these produce. During periods of anxiety and tension, cortisol and adrenaline flood the system in order to deal with the presumed or real threat.

Even more subtle than this are the effects our thoughts can have on other people and situations, although this is a much more intangible phenomenon that is difficult to measure. As many of us learn through practical experience, what we put out into the world seems to come back to us. This can be described as a spiritual law acting out in the present moment. When we emanate positivity, harmony and love in the world, we seem to attract similar people, events and situations into our lives. This does not prevent adverse situations happening, as life is much more complex than that, but the predominant experience of life will be a positive one.

On the other hand, when we project jealousy, envy, hatred and anger into the world, at people and situations, the same negativity will follow us like a shadow. *Karma* dictates that we don't get away with anything, even if we think we do.

Like attracts like. Good follows good. And we all get what we deserve.

The Indian school of philosophy called Vedanta, divides *karma* into three types. The first is what is happening currently (*prarabhda karma*); the second is what is yet to have ripened, or future *karma* (*agami karma*); and the third is from the past (*sanchita karma*).

Past *karma* is a fraction more difficult to fathom, as Eastern traditions believe there are lives before the current life, and that actions from these lives may reach fruition only in later lives. It's impossible to know whether this is fact or fiction, but when bad things happen for no apparent reason, it does give us philosophical solace to think it may be the effect of a past action that we have no recollection of. Life is way too complex to understand the intricacies or creation and all of the resultant effects. Until we've reached a level of experiential knowledge of such matters, we must be guided by wise souls who have gone before us and offered these explanations to us out of their wisdom and compassion.

Sometimes, for no obvious reason at all, everything can become a struggle, or a severe misfortune may occur that makes us wonder about the meaning of life, and why such a bad thing happened. Deaths, tragedies, financial misfortune and relationship breakdowns can all occur as a result of a poorly managed life, but equally, despite the best of intentions and planning, misfortune happens. Bad fortune can be explained in terms of *karma*, but ultimately there may be no good reason that can plausibly be used. It may be a test or a challenge, but still the answer never really seems satisfactory enough. As a surgeon, every day I see young people struck down with cancer. Although I may not always have each person's full life story in front of me in terms of lifestyle, diet and emotional health, on the surface each situation often seems no different from any other.

Life is unpredictable

Despite our best efforts to stay healthy and well, life sometimes seems to have other plans for us. I see it every day in my work.

Last year I diagnosed a life-threatening kidney cancer that was successfully removed; six months later the patient was found to have a moderately aggressive prostate cancer. I didn't know how to give him and his wife the news, except to say that it was rotten luck, or a case of unlucky genetics. He sailed through his prostate-cancer surgery, however, and is now effectively cured of both cancers. Naturally it was a huge emotional rollercoaster ride for both he and his wife, but they've come through stronger, more in love, and with deeper gratitude for every day with their two young children.

A healthy fifty-year-old ambulance offer was diagnosed with kidney cancer that had already spread to his bones. Radiation therapy was administered to his spinal deposit, and I removed his kidney cancer. The spinal deposit grew larger and it was also surgically resected. He remains alive, but with a completely altered approach to life. Each day now is a bonus, and precious. He knows that every day with his wife and children may be his last if the cancer takes over his body.

It's hard to offer an explanation for such sporadic occurrences. Needless to say it offers compelling testimony that we must live our lives to the fullest with no regrets. It doesn't mean that we have to live as if each day was our last—that would a very dour way to exist. At the same time it doesn't mean that we should take a narcissistic or reckless approach either. Instead, the way to be is to make moment-to-moment choices that are in keeping with our intended goals based on what we value most importantly in our lives. 'Don't sweat the small stuff' is about as succinct as it needs to be.

Life is too fickle and unpredictable to take things too seriously and to create unpleasantness in the world. Enjoy the moment. Live life fully, with enthusiasm and vigour. Help other people, and face tests and challenges with your most positive foot forward. Everything else is beyond your control.

Practical step 6

- Identify some of your own inherent cycles with regard to mood and energy levels.
- Identify your attitude to sexuality and how that fits with your overall material and spiritual paths. Is there compatibility or conflict in your relationship?
- Identify three incidents in your life that appeared to be out of the blue that you attribute to fate or *karma* or just a random event.

7

The Cocktail: Joyful Living

When you seek to enjoy a balance of the material and the spiritual, you will need to consider many things, but if you live with awareness, all the different components of life will find their rightful place as neither too important nor too irrelevant. Each aspect needs the correct amount of attention; each has its own specific requirements that only you can ascertain. Physical health, emotional wellbeing, relationships, occupation, money, sex, desires and spiritual trajectory all need to be considered carefully in order to maintain a life of balance.

Now is the time to take your own life into your own hands. Do you want to live your life the way *you* want, or do you want to do the accepted, safe thing? There's no problem in choosing a conservative profession if you feel that path will give you the opportunity to express all your talents. We need our accountants and lawyers and doctors to be brilliant in what they do, because their roles are important, but avoid choosing one of those roles simply because it offers a secure life. You will live your life but you will die of boredom, which is another way of saying your soul will shut down.

As a person who has lived a material and spiritual life, and gone too far in certain directions at times, I am thankful I always had the good fortune and sense to come back to a middle path. I've seen married couples who are deeply in love run into problems when one suddenly falls for a guru, then spends hours in spiritual practices, neglecting the needs of their partner. They may be experiencing spiritual bliss, but at the same time their material life can fall into disarray.

It's a similar situation with children. As fathers, men may find it too easy to slip into the old model of 'mother takes care of the kids', but children need a father too. They grow up so quickly, and the investment in time spent with our children, being good role models, encouraging positive habits and values, and forging healthy relationships is invaluable beyond measure and one of the greatest gifts we can give society. Parents who neglect the needs of their children lose friends for life, and children without guidance miss out on learning from the life wisdom of their parents. Once an opportunity has passed it does not come back again.

The first step is to have thorough self-knowledge. The SWOT analysis mentioned in chapter one is crucial. You need to know what are your strengths, talents and aptitudes, and simultaneously what are your weaknesses and challenges. If your skill set means you will flourish in music or the arts, there's no point trying to forge a career in law or medicine.

Know yourself, know yourself, know yourself. The greatest blessing you will have is to be able to blend your talents with your passions, as well as with the needs of society. This holy trifecta (passion + talent + need) is optimal but is not always available to everyone. For example, you may have the skill and passion for painting with oils, but are unable to make a living from it. In this situation you need to decide whether to alter your lifestyle in order to continue your passion as your main focus, or find an additional source of income.

Alternatively, there's no point trying to pursue professional football as your profession if you can't get into the local under 16Ds. This is where the intellect is required to work out what is your life purpose. What is it that makes you tick? What activity makes you jump out of bed at the crack of dawn, ready to start the day?

This decision involves both head and heart. The heart indicates passion and love of an activity, and the head determines skill and need. It's important to keep certain mental distortions out of this equation, as they will surely lead to an unfulfilling decision.

Fear and greed are two factors that can also lead to wrong decisions being made. Fear sets up a constant state of aversion to engaging in activities that may lead to failure. Fear is limiting, restricting and constricting, and makes you settle for less than you deserve.

Greed, on the other hand, leads to a life of imbalance. Greed for power, money and fame can lead to a path of faulty choices based on what something or someone can do for you. Greed leads to the 'more, bigger, better' mindset. Longer hours of work in order to make more money or gain greater power result in time away from relationships with children and partners, and less attention on health. Everything suffers as a result.

Being healthy is easy, but being vibrant takes a little more care. With attention on physical health and proper food and habits, your body will be fundamentally healthy. Vibrancy takes a different level of consideration. It's up to you as an individual to decide where to place yourself.

There's no time better time than right now to take charge of your life. There's nothing more powerful than being the master of your own destiny. Leave behind those who are holding you back. Your best life may be as a corporate executive, or running the home with efficiency and fulfilment. It doesn't matter what you're doing; it's how you live your life that is most important.

There's nothing more attractive than someone who is happy and passionate about life. They radiate a magnetic energy that people want to be part of. You can call it an aura or a presence. The good news is that living a life of balance is truly possible for every single one of us. Once your awareness has risen to a reasonable level, you'll be able to see things as they really are. By studying the world around you, and observing the pitfalls that others have fallen into, you can navigate through life sensibly and with care.

You can become free of rigid notions about how life should be lived.

You can live with a fluidity that enables you to make free and informed, conscious choices.

You can learn to enjoy all that the world has to offer without strong cravings or attachments, and without becoming a fulltime pleasure seeker.

You can enjoy the pleasures of life, but they will fall into their rightful place, neither suppressed nor chased

You can enjoy a drink or more without worrying that alcohol precludes spirituality.

You can eat meat without feeling that you're a bad person for consuming a living creature.

You can enjoy sex without the idea that it is a sin.

At the same time, you can explore the inner dimensions through any path that appeals to you, realising that no one path carries a monopoly on the truth. As time goes on, you will become less dependent on a particular path, organisation, teaching or guru and come to trust your own inner beacon. You will learn to stabilise your mind no matter what's happening externally, and as that happens you will realise that there's a constant substratum of stillness that's always there behind the scenes.

Once you've learned to calm the mind, there arises a different kind of living that consists of intuition, knowingness and flow. Your inner voice will speak to you loudly and clearly, directing which path to take at any moment. At times it will direct you to travel solo; at times it will require you to take guidance and direction. Removing preconceived notions of what it means to be successful in the material and spiritual domains will free you from projecting things from your own imagination. There is great freedom in this.

Once you get back to basics, it doesn't matter what your external situation is. Whether you're a rich person who lives in a mansion and drives a Ferrari; or a person who enjoys fine wine, meats and pleasures of the body; or a spiritual seeker aiming for enlightenment, it just does not matter. What does matter is being absolutely honest with your own state of being in body, mind, spirit and balance. Only after ascertaining that can you determine how to live your life, and know which choices will be beneficial and which choices will be detrimental.

And, depending on your own unique situation, with awareness you will come to the right blend of balance. Once you strike the balance, it's like a lightbulb going on inside.

Then you will have a life that's free of cravings and aversions, that's inwardly settled yet vibrant, and that's externally equipped to make a positive contribution to everyone and everything around you.

Everyone is entitled to a joyful life. It's up to each one of us to make the best possible choices to enable our outer and inner desires to be fulfilled. With clarity of awareness we all have the ability to make those best possible choices.

It's possible to live a life that encompasses everything that's available on both the material and spiritual planes. Just like a master cocktail maker, your job is to mix the right ingredients in the right proportions, blend them together, enjoy the taste, and know when to start and when to stop.

As a fellow seeker, my advice is to listen to everyone with an open mind and heart, but to keep your intellect sharp as a knife. Be guided by your own judgment and make your choices accordingly. And don't be influenced by those who think *their* way is the only way. A heart that is soft with compassion, blended with an intellect that is razor sharp, along with a mind that is settled and calm, allows for a life of balance, service and joy.

Bruce Springsteen once said at a concert at which his parents were attending,

> *One of you wanted me to be an author, so you could get a little something for yourself.*

The other wanted me to be a lawyer, so you could get a little something for yourself.
What you both didn't realise is that I wanted everything.

Meditation & Martini represents just that path.

Reach for the stars,
and enjoy all that life has to offer.
Be prepared for a few bumps along the way,
and keep smiling.

As you explore life in its totality, I wish you all the best in health and wellness.